Growing Bean

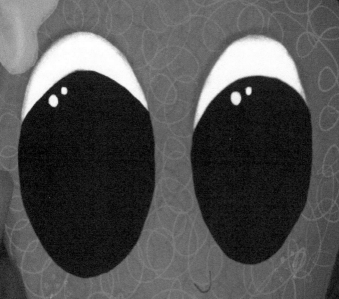

Katy Delaney

illustrated by
Rachael Laurie

Published in the United Kingdom by:

Blue Falcon Publishing
The Mill, Pury Hill Business Park,
Alderton Road, Towcester
Northamptonshire
NN12 7LS
Email: books@bluefalconpublishing.co.uk
Web: www.bluefalconpublishing.co.uk

A CIP record of this book is available from the British Library.

First printed March 2022

ISBN 978-1912765430

To my Mum & Dad
For always believing in me and forever supporting
me. My Husband Aaron for his constant love and
support and my very own 3 Growing Beans Lanais,
Noah & Parker who without them this book may
never have been.
-K.D

Growing Bean

by **Katy Delaney**

illustrated by Rachael Laurie

I still can't feel you wriggle
but I know that you are there.
Swimming safely in your home,
I rub my tum with care.

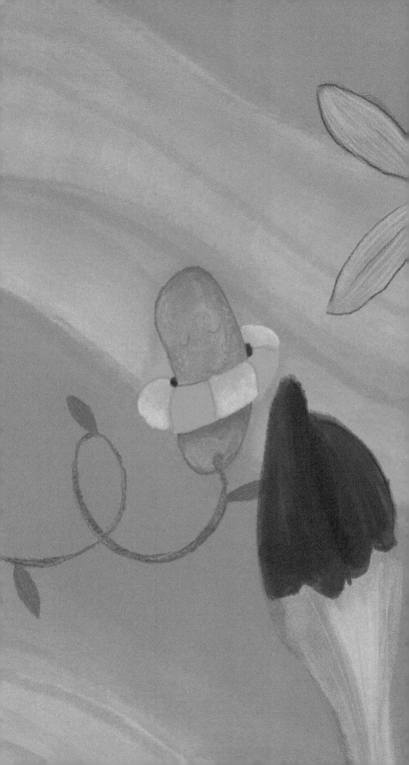

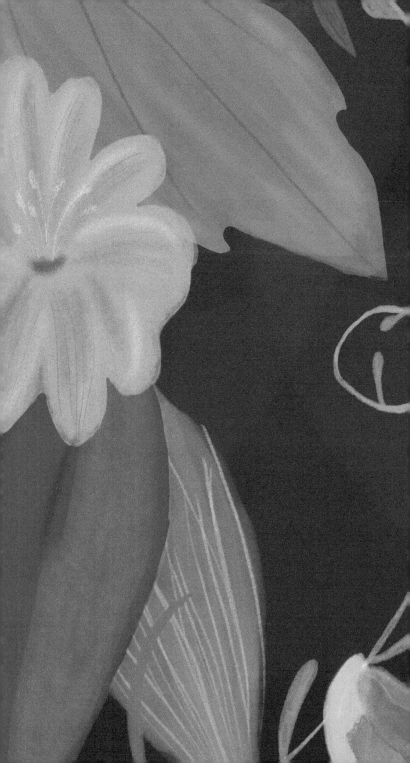

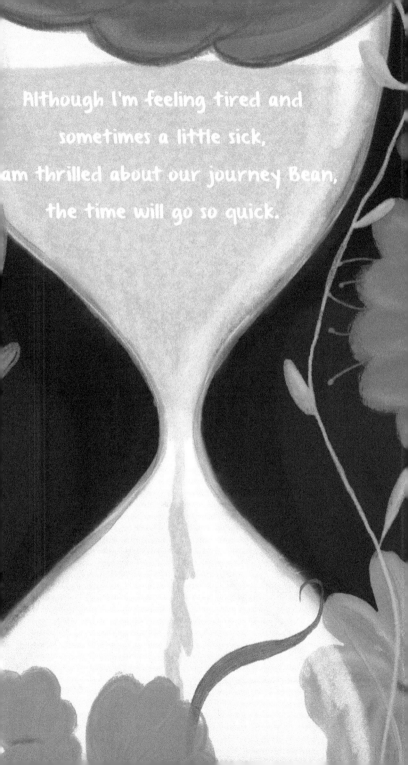

Although I'm feeling tired and
sometimes a little sick,
am thrilled about our journey Bean,
the time will go so quick.

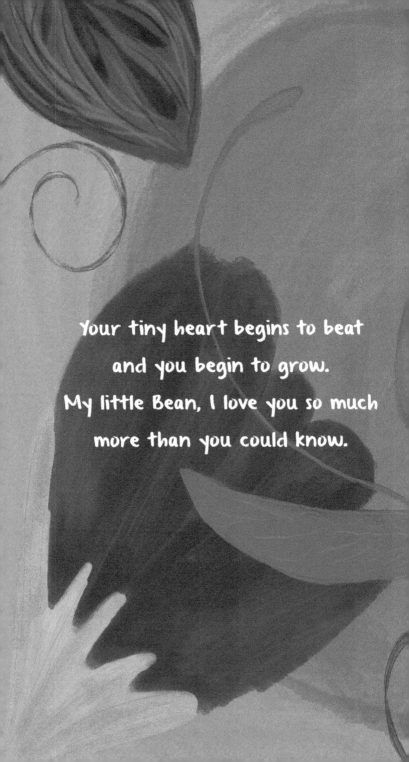

Your tiny heart begins to beat
and you begin to grow.
My little Bean, I love you so much
more than you could know.

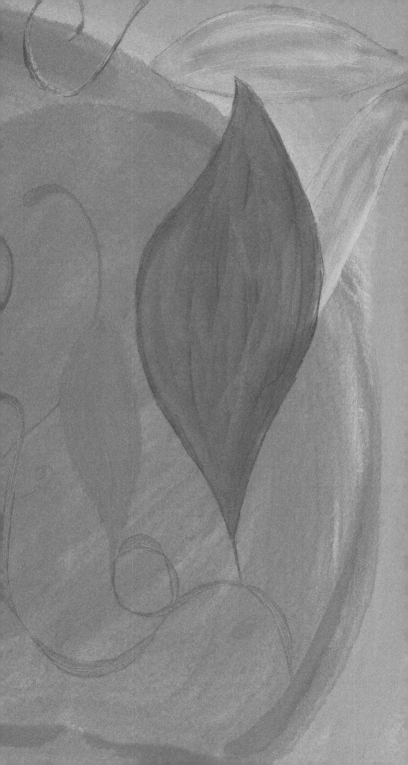

I get to hear your heart beat now
and see you on the scan,
Oh, how much I love those photos
I've become your biggest fan.

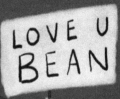

A wave of flutters deep inside:

my little Bean's in flight.

I can feel you say hello to me

and make my tummy tight.

Keep on growing, little Bean,

until your day is due.

I shall cross off the days my Bean;

I can't wait to meet you.

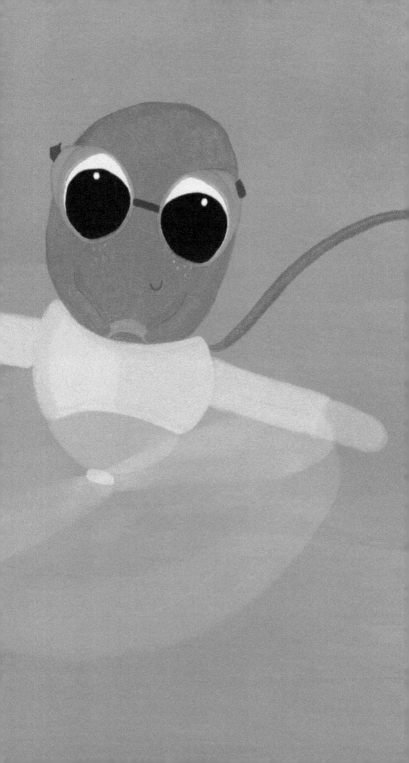

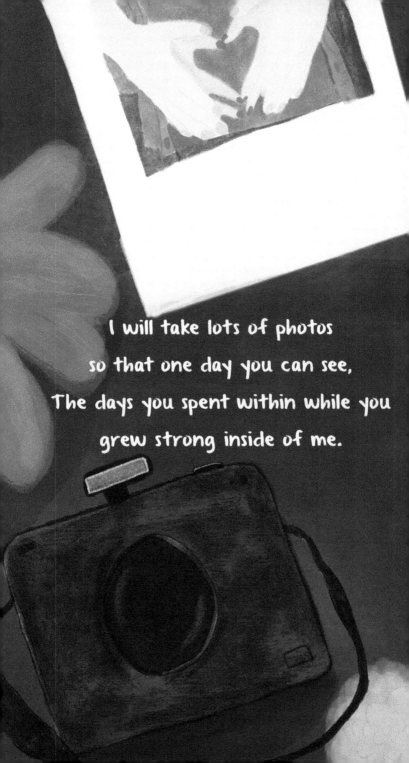

I will take lots of photos
so that one day you can see,
The days you spent within while you
grew strong inside of me.

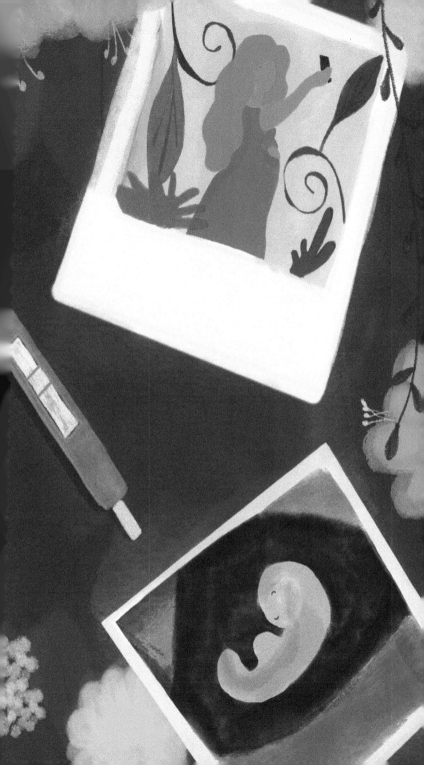

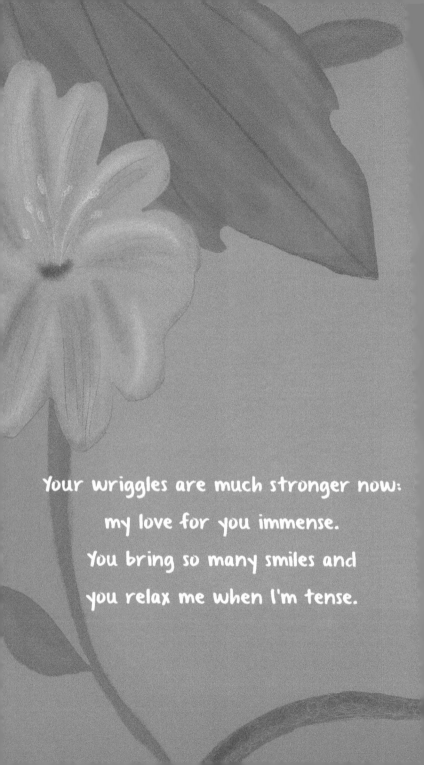

Your wriggles are much stronger now:
my love for you immense.
You bring so many smiles and
you relax me when I'm tense.

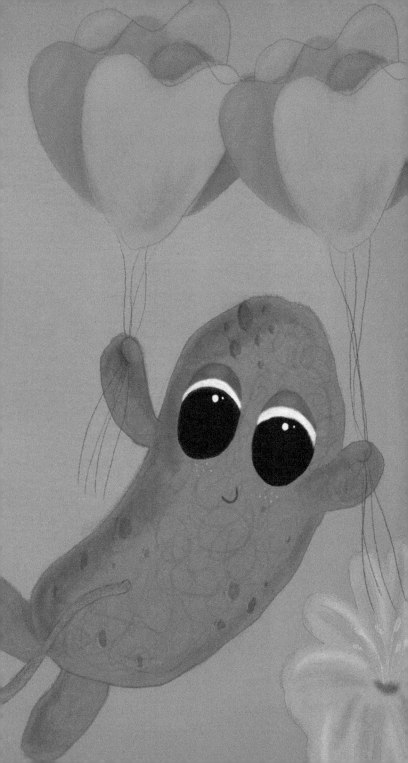

I cannot wait
to meet you,
my little growing
Bean.
To see that little
face of yours,
the cutest face
I've seen.
Until that day
comes,
I'll keep you safe
and warm.
You are content
inside of me,
kicking up a
storm.

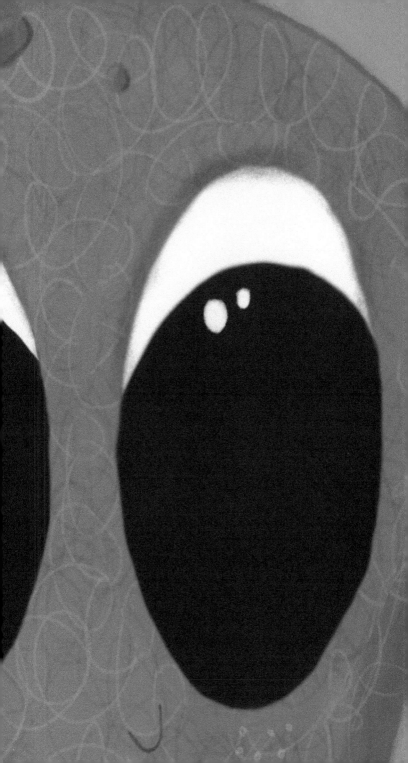

Your kicks are hard and fast now;

I'm bursting at the seams.

I feel your foot, your elbow,

my poor ribs that you tag team!

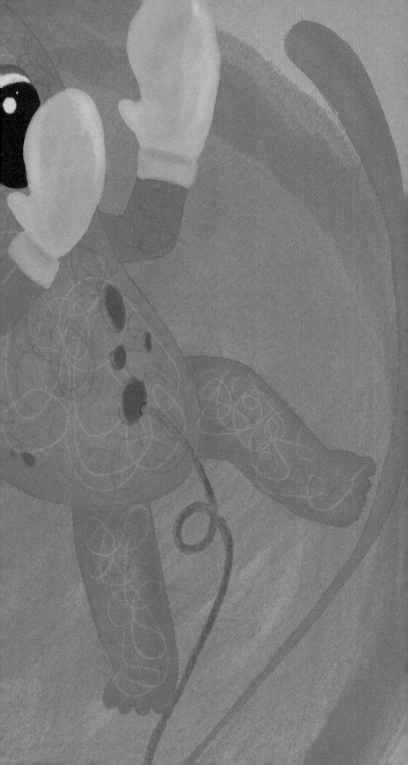

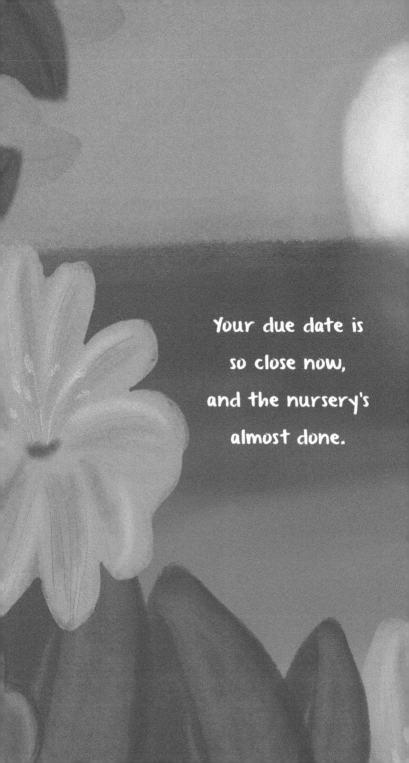

Your due date is
so close now,
and the nursery's
almost done.

Little Bean,
we will soon know -
a daughter
or a son?

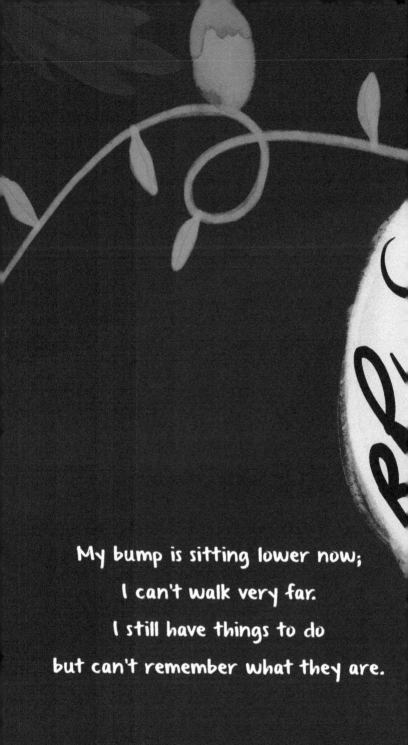

My bump is sitting lower now;
I can't walk very far.
I still have things to do
but can't remember what they are.

teeth

CLEAN

lunch

Toilet Break

Relax

Shower

DRINK

You know the sound
of my voice now,
however could you not?
I've read this book to you
most nights;
you knew when I forgot.

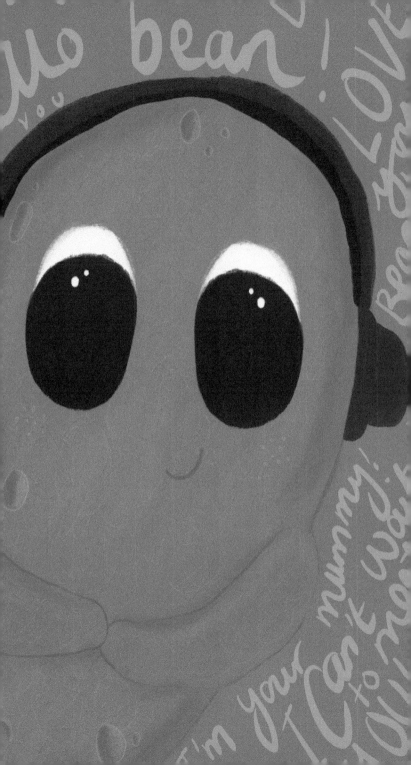

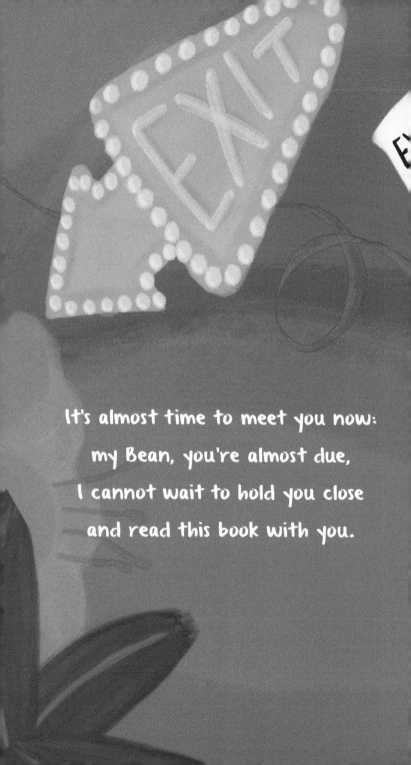

It's almost time to meet you now:
my Bean, you're almost due,
I cannot wait to hold you close
and read this book with you.

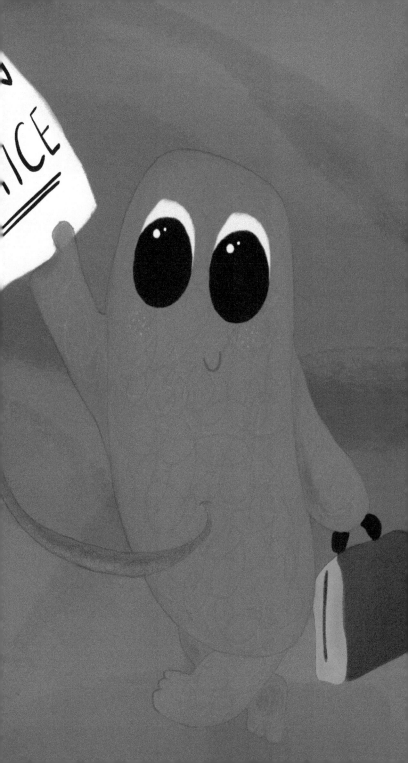

Introducing Our Little Bean

Name:

Born on: Day: Date: Month:

Time:

Where:

Weight:

Length:

Hair Colour:

Eye Colour:

Who was there?

(Space for photo)

A Letter to Our Bean on your 1st Birthday
(Space for parents to handwrite letter)

Lightning Source UK Ltd.
Milton Keynes UK
UKHW020427030322
399402UK00001B/1